Distribution, publication, and copying in any form are prohibited and subject to damages.

TEN HYPNOSES

Copying, publishing, and sharing with third parties are only permitted with the written consent of the author. Please observe the notes on copyright and usage.

Distribution, publication, and copying in any form are prohibited and subject to damages.

Copying, publishing, and sharing with third parties are only permitted with the written consent of the author. Please observe the notes on copyright and usage.

Distribution, publication, and copying in any form are prohibited and subject to damages.

Ingo Michael Simon

TEN HYPNOSES

38
FEAR OF INJECTIONS

Copying, publishing, and sharing with third parties are only permitted with the written consent of the author. Please observe the notes on copyright and usage.

Distribution, publication, and copying in any form are prohibited and subject to damages.

© 2024 Ingo Michael Simon
All rights reserved.
Independently published
www.ingosimon.com

Important Notes for Urgent Attention:

The contents of this book are based on the practical experiences of the author with hypnosis applications and psychotherapy in a trance state. Although the author has strived for the utmost care, errors or misunderstandings in the presentation cannot be completely excluded. Therapeutic work with people and the application of hypnosis are solely the responsibility of the hypnotist. It cannot be ruled out that parts of this book may be misunderstood or that the application of a presented procedure may cause an undesirable reaction in the client. The author also assumes no co-responsibility if work with a client is carried out with reference to the statements in this book.

The Author:

Ingo Michael Simon studied psychology and education and is a hypnotherapist with practices in southwestern Germany and Switzerland. With the help of hypnosis-supported psychotherapy, he primarily treats people with persistent psychological conditions. His practice focuses on anxiety disorders, pathological compulsions, and psychosomatic illnesses. His therapeutic offerings mainly include classical and modern hypnosis applications and the dreamland therapy he developed himself.

Copying, publishing, and sharing with third parties are only permitted with the written consent of the author. Please observe the notes on copyright and usage.

Distribution, publication, and copying in any form are prohibited and subject to damages.

INTRODUCTION — 6

COPYRIGHT AND USAGE — 8

HYPNOSIS 1 — 10

HYPNOSIS 2 — 15

HYPNOSIS 3 — 20

HYPNOSIS 4 — 26

HYPNOSIS 5 — 31

HYPNOSIS 6 — 36

HYPNOSIS 7 — 40

HYPNOSIS 8 — 46

HYPNOSIS 9 — 52

HYPNOSIS 10 — 57

ALL TITLES IN THE SERIES — 63

Copying, publishing, and sharing with third parties are only permitted with the written consent of the author. Please observe the notes on copyright and usage.

Introduction

The series "Ten Hypnoses" is very well known in Germany, Austria, and Switzerland as a collection of texts for therapeutic work and is used by numerous psychotherapeutic practices, doctors, therapists, coaches, and other helping professionals. I am pleased to now be able to offer these texts in other countries as well.

Most therapists have their own methods for inducing and deepening trance as well as for exiting trance. Therefore, I have focused on the main part of the hypnosis. The texts in this book can be integrated as the main part into any hypnosis process. The texts in this collection use various hypnosis techniques. I will not explain these in detail, as I assume that users have the appropriate training. It is also not necessary to understand the exact structure or functioning of the different parts. The texts can simply be read aloud, and they will have their effect.

Decide for yourself which text best suits your client or patient at any given time. You can also combine passages from different texts. It is not about using all ten hypnoses in sequence. It is a selection of possibilities.

I want to emphasize that books cannot replace therapy. Psychotherapy or other therapeutic treatments involve much more. A careful diagnosis is the necessary basis for deciding on the use of methods, including whether hypnosis or one of my texts should be used. Even in this case, preparatory discussions, follow-up discussions during the session, and of course, a therapeutic concept for the sequence of sessions and the content approaches are essential parts of therapy. This cannot and should not be achieved with a collection of texts.

In any case, I wish you much success in your work and I am pleased if my text templates can contribute in a small way.

Ingo Michael Simon

Copyright and Usage

Copying, publishing, and sharing with third parties is prohibited and only permitted with the written consent of the author. Please observe the following copyright and usage guidelines.

This work has been carefully crafted and created to the best of the author's knowledge and personal experience. It comprises text templates and application guidelines for professional hypnosis sessions. The author is a licensed psychotherapist with extensive experience in psychotherapy, coaching, and personal training using hypnotic techniques and methods. Nevertheless, the author and the publisher assume no liability for the accuracy of information, instructions, and advice, nor for any typographical errors. The author and publisher accept no responsibility or liability for the application of these texts and recommendations with clients or patients, nor for any potential consequences or unexpected reactions. It is expressly noted that the application of therapeutic and advisory techniques and formulations lies solely and entirely within the responsibility of the practitioner. This also applies to adherence to the boundaries of legally regulated medical and therapeutic practices. The fact that a book containing action proposals is freely available for sale does not imply that its application with clients or patients is permitted for everyone.

Hypnosis 1

You want to put an end to your fear today, because it is time to really let it go ... ... You have decided ... ... You want to finally release the fear, because it no longer serves any purpose ... ... You are familiar with the fear of needles and injections, but that is now in the past ... ... It is over ... ... It is truly over, because today you are making a change ... ... You are shifting your thoughts to relaxation ... ... Relaxation with needles and injections ... ... You are shifting your feelings towards relaxation ... ... Relaxation with needles and injections ... ... You are making the shift ... ... You have already made the shift ... ... You have already taken this step of change internally ... ... You have already taken this step towards freedom internally ... ... Today, you take it for your waking life ... ... From today on, you can also handle needles and injections with ease while awake ... ... As soon as you are fully awake again, you will be free ... ...

When your mind thinks about the fear of injections, you quickly realize that it is unfounded ... ... It was an exaggerated fear that you can now influence with your thoughts ... ... You can change it ... ... Because ultimately, it is always thoughts that lead to exaggerated fears ... ... because at some point, you judged a concern or uncertainty too harshly ... ... So first, you change your thinking ... ... So, here and now, you make it clear to yourself that a small needle cannot harm you at all ... ... that a small needle does not even hurt ... ... It just gives you a small pinch ... ... So, you simply think ... ... Needles do not matter to me at all ... ... You might still doubt this, but in a few moments it will be so ... ... Maybe it is already the case, because in trance, in this beautiful relaxation, needles really do not matter to you at all ... ...

You feel the calmness of your body, because you are now in this beautiful state of deep calm ... ... truly deep calm ... ... Now, it is also easy to recognize that your body is in complete safety ... ... You are completely safe here ... ... Nothing can happen to you or your body now ... ... and now you can also imagine that a small prick is no problem at all for your body ... ... A small sting is just as insignificant ... ... Surely, you have been bitten by a mosquito before and felt a little prick ... ... no big deal ... ... actually not a problem at all ... ... Your body easily handles it ... ... Your body can now adjust even more to experiencing a small prick as insignificant … … to considering the prick of a small needle as insignificant … … insignificant needles … … insignificant pricks … … insignificant little sting … …

Body and feelings are closely connected … … A calm and relaxed body helps you to be calm internally as well … … It even makes you automatically calm inside … … You are experiencing that right now … … Because your body is relaxed … … relaxed in deep trance … … you are also relaxed inside … … relaxed in your feelings … … You feel calmness and serenity within you … … you can now even think calmly about injections … … and still remain calm and serene … … because your body is helping you … … because your body is helping you now and will help you in your waking state as well … … And now it is completely clear to you that your body hardly registers a small needle prick … … Your body smiles at a small needle prick … … And when you get an injection, it is again the case that your body can laugh about it … … It hardly feels it, and it does not care … … and this feeling is now clearly passed on to your thoughts by your body … … Then it also does not matter to you in your thoughts to see a needle … …

There are even more connections between body and feelings ... ... There is the special connection between action, body, and feelings ... ... Just as your body sensations influence your emotions, so your actions influence your body and therefore your feelings as well ... ... It is very simple ... ... At the beginning of the trance, you experienced how you calmed down through actions ... ... You made yourself comfortable ... ... You closed your eyes ... ... and you breathed slowly and evenly ... ... You are still doing that ... ... and exactly that helped your body to enter this beautiful state of deep relaxation and to stay there ... ... This also works in your everyday life ... ... Conscious calm breathing calms your body ... ... keeps your heartbeat calm ... ... and as a result, you feel emotionally relaxed as well ... ... free from any fear and full of peace ... ... free from fear and full of peace ... ... peace that makes you serene ... ... and needles do not matter to you ... ... Needles are completely indifferent to you ... ... Needles are truly indifferent to you ... ...

You have come much closer to your goal today ... ... because you have already changed your basic attitude towards needles and injections ... ... You have changed more than you might think ... ... You have realized that it was a completely exaggerated fear that had taken hold of you ... ... You have adjusted your thoughts, have taken to heart the thought that tells you ... ... Needles do not matter to me at all ... ... first as an idea, as a wish ... ... But today, in trance, this wish has sunk deeper and become a truth ... ... Your body has remained calm ... ... You have remained calm inside ... ... calm in the thought of needles and injections ... ... and this calmness remains ... ... because you will always be able to stay calm and remain calm with injections ... ... Needles do not matter to you at all ... ... You just keep breathing naturally ... ... calmly breathing in and out ... ... free from fear and full of peace ... ... truly free from fear and full of peace ... ...

Hypnosis 2

Today, you want to let go of your fear of injections ... ... You want to be able to give injections or set up IV lines with ease again ... ... You used to do it before ... ... You have given many injections/set up many lines before, and it was easy for you ... ... You did it naturally ... ... It was routine for you, and it will become routine again ... ...   Giving injections/setting up lines will become natural for you again ... ... You can do it ... ...   It really works for you because you used to be able to give injections/set up lines with ease ... ... Today is the day you rediscover your ease and confidence ... ... You can do it ... ...

You remember the time when you handled needles or injections naturally ... ... It was a pleasant and easy routine for you ... ... You could do it, so you can still do it ... ...   You remember your old and good routine with injections/IVs ... ... This reawakens this stable, learned routine within you ... ... and the calmness ... ...   You make it clear to yourself that you really could do it and remained completely calm ... ... It will be that way again because you are reactivating your own competence ... ... You already have it ... ... So today, you are actually using your own experience ... ... your own competence, because you do not need to learn anything new ... ... You do not need to build new courage or calmness ... ... You awaken the courage you once had and still have within you ... ... You awaken the self-confidence you once had and still have within you ... ... Now ... ... You could do it, and you can do it ... ... You could really do it, and you can really do it ... ... You can do it today ... ... You end the fear of needles and remain calm ... ... Now ... ...

We work step by step ... ... You know this from your own work ... ... You also proceed step by step there ... ... So, you do it the same way here ... ... You have already taken the first steps ... ... You have already taken important steps ... ... You have already reached the trance and awakened your memory of your own competence and calmness ... ... Competence and calmness with injections and needles ... ... You had them, and you still have them ... ... With that, you have already taken some important steps and are on a very good path ... ... on your path to success ... ... Now we neutralize the needles ... ... Imagine a needle or injection lying on a table because it has already been administered ...

... It no longer has any significance, everything is done ... ... The needle, the injection is meaningless ... ... It is already done ... ... Everything has already been done ... ... The needle is now meaningless ... ... A used needle or injection is discarded because it has become useless ... ... The needle is disposed of ... ... You no longer need it ... ... This is just an imagination, just a fantasy ... ... But it is also more than that ... ... because now needles are already neutralized ... ... Needles have already become truly insignificant deep within you ... ... Very good, because needles are now indeed completely meaningless ... ... You can take the next step ... ...

For the next step, imagine again a syringe or cannula on a table ... ... It keeps you calm because needles are now neutral ... ... Now, in this trance, needles are truly neutral ... ... very good ... ... Imagine that you will use this needle shortly, you will use it on a patient ... ... That is very simple ... ... That is really simple now ... ... Using the needle or syringe is now, in this imagination, very simple ... ... That is how it used to be as well ... ... You even enjoyed doing it, and above all, you did it naturally ... ... Needles were a good tool for you ... ... Needles are now a good tool again ... ...

You can do important things with them, and you enjoy doing them … … You find needles for IVs … … cannulas and injections good again … … Even the thought of actually using them, you find good … … really good … …

You are a therapist (nurse, medical assistant, etc.), and you have done something very special today … … You have treated yourself in just a few steps today … … You have eliminated your fear of needles … … You have really successfully treated yourself here and today in just a few but correct steps … … You have regained your old naturalness … … You have achieved your goal, approached needles and injections again … … You allow yourself to be happy that you have achieved this … … You even allow yourself to be proud … … proud that you faced this fear and eliminated it … … Everything is good … … In your waking everyday life, you will naturally use needles again or give injections … … naturally … …

Today, you have successfully treated yourself … … Perhaps you are already looking forward to experiencing once again being completely free and relaxed the next time you handle needles or injections … … You feel safe and free … … From now on, you feel safe and free in dealing with needles ... ... You really and truly feel free and safe again ... ... and with each day, you feel more and more that dealing with needles and injections is very simple for you ... ... really simple for you ... ...

Hypnosis 3

You have decided to let go of the fear of needles and injections today … … You have even decided to let go of these fears once and for all … … That is a good decision because you know that these fears no longer make sense … … You know there is no danger and that an injection causes nothing more than a small pinch … … that nothing can happen to you … … Your mind knows this, and that is why your mind has also decided to let go of the fear in this hypnosis today and replace it with the feeling of relaxation … … because only one of these two feelings can be present … … Fear or relaxation … … And you choose relaxation … …

… … You succeed in trance … … It succeeds in this hypnosis because under hypnosis you can change things that are not so easily influenced in waking life … … But now … … already relaxed and calm inside, you can achieve so much more … …

Now, breathe calmly and evenly and consciously feel your body … … Notice the contact with the surface and feel that your body is being supported … … Now let your breath flow consciously ... ... Imagine your breath flowing through your entire body ... ... into your lungs and from there deep into your abdomen ... ... and finally into your arms and legs ... ... This brings your body even more into a state of calm ... ... This allows you to relax even deeper and feel your body better ... ... you can perceive it more consciously ... ... because it is now all about your body feeling ... ... Your body has come to rest, but there are always certain areas of the body that are especially calm and relaxed ... ...

... ... Simply move your thoughts along your body and find a spot that feels particularly calm and relaxed ... ... Perhaps your feet feel particularly calm because they no longer have to carry any weight ... ... or your legs are particularly relaxed ... ... It could also be that your back is the most comfortable area ... ... or another spot that you find ... ... Now, find the spot on your body that feels the best ... ... the most comfortable ... ...

... ... Wherever it is, now direct your full awareness to this relaxed and comfortable spot ... ... If your entire body feels good and you cannot decide, just choose a spot that spontaneously comes to mind ... ... and direct your awareness there ... ...

... ... Now keep breathing calmly and evenly and let even more calmness settle in ... ... This spot on your body now relaxes even deeper ... ... very good ... ... That is exactly right ... ... Feel the relaxation very consciously ... ... Let it become very clear in your perception ... ... very good ... ... This is really good because now you can do something special ... ... Now you can ensure that injections are easy to handle ... ... that you remain calm when you receive an injection ... ...

... ... Now find the spot on your body where you will receive an injection ... ... You know where that is ... ... Likewise, you can choose a spot where you once received an injection ... ... Your body remembers it because our body stores everything that happens in our life ... ... Now you are relaxed ... ... Now you are in trance, so you can remember and remain calm ... ... Find the injection spot and direct your awareness there ... ... The memory of the injection is there ... ... The expectation of the injection is also there ... ... But you are calm now ... ...

... ... And in this calm, you can achieve even more ... ... You can connect the two spots, so that now and always, as much calmness as possible flows from the calm spot to the injection spot ... ... That way, fear does not even arise ... ... So, now imagine a connecting line between the two spots you have found ... ... a line from the comfortable spot to the injection spot on your body ... ... Imagine it like an arrow pointing from the calm, comfortable spot to the injection spot ... ... and sending calmness there ... ... The memory of calmness and serenity is stored at the comfortable spot ... ... of the calmness you are feeling now, and now you are truly feeling calmness ... ... And this memory of calmness now flows to the injection spot ... ... Now ... ... And the injection spot learns from this calmness ... ... Your body learns for you to remain calm and feel only calmness at the injection spot ... ... Now ... ... Now ... ...

... ... Focus on this image, on this idea ... ... More and more calmness and relaxation flow to the injection spot on your body ... ... more and more calmness ... ... This way, in this moment, this spot on your body also becomes a calm zone ... ... This way, in this moment, the injection spot on your body truly becomes a calm zone ... ... Imagine an arrow as a connecting line between the two areas ... ... The arrow points from the comfortable spot to the injection spot ... ...

… … That is how it should be … … Imagine it … … The more you succeed in seeing this arrow in your mind's eye, the more calmness also flows to the injection spot and stays there … … This creates a new memory in your body … … the memory of calmness and relaxation at the injection spot … … this creates a new connection in your body … … The connection of calmness and injections is established … … The connection of calmness and needles is established … … and as soon as you come into contact with a needle or injection, your body will again send calmness and relaxation to the spot where you receive the injection … … just like now … … exactly like now … … Your body has understood this … … Your body has learned this …

You may also wonder how you can best maintain this … … what you can do to ensure that this connection between calmness and injections truly remains long-term … … It is quite simple … … it is actually easier than you might think … … because your body has learned this for you … … And every time you draw an arrow between the spot you found as comfortable today and the spot of the injection, your body sends calmness and relaxation to the injection, and you can ignore it … …

… … So, you can build this image for yourself a few more times … … But soon, you won't even think about injections anymore … … They will soon be completely indifferent to you … … Injections are indifferent to you … …

Hypnosis 4

You are determined to let go of the fear of needles today ... ... You know that the best way to do this is through deep, inner trust ... ... and so today, you align yourself with this deep trust ... ... because as soon as you can feel this trust within you, the fear automatically fades away ... ... because trust is no longer compatible with fear ... ... Trust sends you the feeling of security ... ... gives you the certainty of safety ... ... Feelings are often fixed thoughts ... ... Thoughts that have become so strong that they have turned into feelings ... ... So, it is also thoughts that free you from burdensome feelings ... ... good and constructive thoughts that create a new truth within you ... ... the new truth of trust ... ... and fear fades away ... ... And in place of the fear, more and more trust takes over ... ... Trust in the fact that you are safe ... ... Trust that you can and will remain calm even with needles and injections ... ... Trust in yourself ... ... deep trust in yourself ... ... real, deep trust in yourself ... ...

Imagine you are surrounded by beautiful light ... ... A very pleasant, white, and warm light surrounds you ... ... And you slowly become one with the light … … Your body is embraced by the white light … … It gently and softly penetrates your skin and fills you from within … … White light, which is very pleasant and warm, gently penetrates your skin … … and flows deep inside you … … Your whole body is flooded with white light … … and step by step, you become one with the light … … You completely merge with the white light … … You blend with the light … … It radiates out from you … … and slowly, all your thoughts disappear into the light … … Nothing is important anymore … … You just dive deeper and deeper into the image of the light … … completely surrounded and filled with light … … and it becomes quieter and quieter within you … … You feel freer and lighter … … Then the light steps out of your body and surrounds you like a pillar … … You are in a pillar of light … … and you still feel connected to the white light that surrounds you … … because a part of the light has remained within you … … Then you notice that the pillar of light is like a curtain that surrounds you … … a curtain of pure light … … a dense curtain of white light, which is very pleasant and warm … …

The curtain of light slowly opens, the long, dense curtain of white light slowly slides aside ... ... The curtain of light that surrounds you opens wider and wider ... ... and you look out from the light ... ... You look directly at a glass wall in front of you ... ... There, in thick letters, a declaration of trust is written ... ... It says ... ...

I let go of all fears and worries, and I trust in the deep calmness and safety within me.

... [Read the affirmation slowly and a little louder than the previous text to emphasize it. Then, pause for about 30 seconds before continuing.] ...

These words of trust work deeply within you ... ... They originated there and unfold their effect there ... ... because they express your belief ... ... your new belief ... ... You had this mindset before ... ... before you knew fear of needles or injections ... ... and today, you look at this belief within you once again ... ... and with that, this belief, this affirmation becomes the new belief within you ... ... the belief and conviction that you have rediscovered today ... ... Because deep within you, it was always like this ... ... Deep within you, you always believed this ... ... Deep within you, you were always convinced of self-confidence and trust … … and this trust helps you today to truly let go of the fear of needles and injections … … to hand it over to the past … … and to be truly free … …

These words, which you can see and read again behind the curtain of light, work deep within you and you can confirm them again … …

I let go of all fears and worries, and I trust in the deep calmness and safety within me.

… [Read the affirmation slowly and a little louder than the previous text to emphasize it. Then, pause for about 30 seconds before continuing.] …

… … Now, allow yourself to simply rest and let the effect of these words unfold … … You do not have to do anything for it … … You do not need to exert yourself … … It is enough that you are here and allow the calmness to settle in … … Breathe calmly and evenly … … because with the flow of your breath, the effect of the words flows deeper into your being … …

Very good … … Every day, you can repeat these words, this affirmation … … and with each repetition, it helps you to let go of the fear and embrace trust ... ... the deep trust that lies within you ... ... that has always lain within you ... ... The fear ends and trust begins ... ... You can start each day with your affirmation and end it with it as well ... ... You can make every day a day of trust with your declaration of trust ... ... every day ... ... every single day ... ...

Hypnosis 5

You want to let go of the fear today ... ... You want to let go of the fear of needles today ... ... You want to let go of the fear of injections today ... ... You have decided, and today you will succeed ... ... Today, you succeed in letting go of the fear and feeling good about it ... ... You have focused entirely on getting this done ... ... and now you can concentrate even more on losing the fear ... ... because now you are in trance, and in trance, you can concentrate better ... ... In trance, you can better communicate your desires and goals to your subconscious ... ... Your subconscious helps you when it is sure that you want it ... ... So, you talk to your subconscious ... ... You talk to your subconscious and, in doing so, you tell yourself what you want to feel and think ... ... You decide what is allowed ... ... You say ... ...

... ... I let go of the fear of needles and injections ... ... because I have the firm goal of deciding for myself what is allowed ... ...

… … I let go of the fear of needles and injections … … because I am sure that I am doing something good for myself … …

… … I let go of the fear of needles and injections … … because it is clear to me that it is an exaggerated assessment … …

… … I let go of the fear of needles and injections … … because I know that injections can often help me and are important … …

… … I can do this … … Yes, I can do this … …

… … I fill my mind with positive and beautiful thoughts … … because positive thoughts help me to take on and overcome any challenge … …

… … I fill my mind with positive and beautiful thoughts … … because I know that every fear dissolves into positive thoughts … …

… … I fill my mind with positive and beautiful thoughts … … because with them, I can calmly look at or even receive an injection … …

… … I fill my mind with positive and beautiful thoughts … … because I prefer to think positively and feel good … …

… … I can do this … … Yes, I can do this … …

… … For my body, a small prick is just a light pinch … … and that is why my body also remains calm with an injection … …

… … For my body, a small prick is just a light pinch … … and that is why an injection almost feels like a light tickle … …

… … For my body, a small prick is just a light pinch … … and that is why I do not care about injections … …

… … For my body, a small prick is just a light pinch … … and that is why I let go of the old fear of needles and injections … …

… … I can do this … … Yes, I can do this … …

… … I am and remain in an inner state of calm … … because I have recognized that everything is okay and there is nothing to fear … …

… … I am and remain in an inner state of calm … … because I know that an injection really helps me … …

… … I am and remain in an inner state of calm … … because I always stay calm when I receive help … …

… … I am and remain in an inner state of calm … … because I want it that way and because I have decided so … …

… … I can do this … … Yes, I can do this … …

… … I breathe calmly and evenly when I see an injection … … because that helps me to become calm and trust … …

… … I breathe calmly and evenly when I see an injection … … because I know that calm breathing calms my body … …

… … I breathe calmly and evenly when I see an injection … … because I know that calm breathing also calms me inside … …

… … I breathe calmly and evenly when I see an injection … … because with it, I overcome the fear, let it go, and am truly free … …

… … I can do this … … Yes, I can do this … … [Now, remain silent for about 30 seconds.] …

Now, continue to breathe calmly and evenly … … Experience now that calm breathing keeps you calm inside … … Here and today, it works … … and what works here and today works always and everywhere … … You have adjusted yourself internally … … You have distanced the fear and become freer … … Injections are indifferent to you … … You have let go of the fear … … And every day, you let go of all fearful thoughts … … just like today … … just like today … …

Hypnosis 6

You want to let go of the fear of needles and injections today … … You know that there were experiences and memories that actually had nothing to do with needles and injections, but over time led to this fear … … You know that with this fear, something is breaking out … … Something is finding its way out … … Feelings that want to be seen … … Memories that can be considered and processed … … They have nothing to do with needles … … They were emotional pricks that you once received … … But the fear can be changed because it is not necessary to have it … … Your subconscious can help you, your deep inner self … … because you are now ready to accept and process what appears as fear … … you are now ready to accept what lies within you … … So, you turn to an instance that can help you … … an instance that you can best believe in because it can really help you … … My words are your words … … You say … …

Dear subconscious / Dear inner helper / Dear guardian angel … … Please help me to let go of the fear of needles and injections again because it has not always accompanied me ... ... I know that it is not the needles and injections that scare me ... ... I know that it was the many pricks of life ... ... the events of my life that were like many small needle pricks ... ... I simply moved on from many of them, continued on, and did not deal with them enough ... ... So, it has come to pass that needles evoke this fear in me ... ... Dear subconscious / Dear inner helper / Dear guardian angel ... ... I am sure that with your help and under your guidance, I can let go of this fear again to deal with the pricks that it is really about ... ...

Dear subconscious / Dear inner helper / Dear guardian angel ... ... I also ask you to help me develop a good feeling when I see a needle or a syringe ... ... After letting go of the fear, I can succeed in feeling good when it comes to injections ... ... I can feel good with your help because I know that the fear has nothing to do with the needle ... ... I know that it only shows up there, but its origin lies deeper ... ... Dear subconscious / Dear inner helper / Dear guardian angel ... ... I trust your guidance ... ... I know that you can guide and help me ... ... I also know that it is I who must allow this help ... ... and I am ready for that ... ... I am ready to accept what is really there ... ... I can and want to recognize, with your support, what really frightened me ... ... Whatever it may be, I accept it and deal with it ... ...

Dear subconscious / Dear inner helper / Dear guardian angel ... ... I ask for your support in being truly mindful and understanding your hints and signals to me ... ... I want to consciously perceive and accept everything that rises from the depths of my feelings because I know that my own feelings and memories cannot harm me ... ... Only repressing these feelings and memories can cause harm ... ... and with your help ... ... Dear subconscious / Dear inner helper / Dear guardian angel ... ... I succeed even better in accepting my own feelings and dealing with them constructively ... ... I firmly trust that it will succeed ... ... and I am sure that I can and will free myself from the fear of needles for good ... ...

Dear subconscious / Dear inner helper / Dear guardian angel ... ... Please be by my side so that I can always accept myself and always encounter myself again ... ... Even if the fear should show itself again, I want to accept it and deal with it ... ... I am aware that it is not the fight against feelings that can help, but only accepting and dealing with them ... ... When I deal with the fear and with all my feelings

… … respect and understand them, then I respect myself … … and then the fear will leave me the quickest … … Dear subconscious / Dear inner helper / Dear guardian angel … … Please also be by my side if I do not lose the fear as quickly … … if it may take longer than I want … … and if I become impatient with the fear and with myself … … Help me to still accept myself well … … I also trust in your support for that … … I trust in your help and your guidance … …

Now, let these words, which are like your own, flow deep into your inner self … … Breathe calmly and evenly and remain calm and relaxed … … because in calmness, the words you have heard, and that a part of yourself has said, can work deeply and free you now … … free you from fear … … You become free inside … … You truly become free inside … … Now … …

Hypnosis 7

Instructions for Execution

This method is a variation of a technique from behavioral therapy. In the so-called systematic desensitization, stimuli that trigger a fear response are collected. In the case of needle phobia, these are stimuli related to the injection situation. These triggers are first sorted into a fear hierarchy, starting with the stimulus that causes only a little fear, up to the one that triggers the greatest fear, in the case of needle phobia, certainly the puncturing with the needle. Step by step, the fear triggers are then presented and relaxation exercises are used to counteract the fear that may arise. Ideally, the low-threshold stimuli, with which one begins, do not trigger fear. Due to the experience that fear-triggering stimuli do not actually trigger fear, the fear threshold is gradually raised. This means that even significant fear triggers eventually lose their terror and no longer cause fear or at least less fear. In trance, we work by identifying some stimuli that are similar to the greatest fear trigger and using them surrounded by relaxation suggestions. Step by step, we approach the greatest fear trigger. Starting with the puncturing of the skin with the injection needle, I have chosen pressure on the injection site as a stimulus, which I first apply as a light pressure with the finger, then as firmer pressure, in a third round with a pen (with the tip retracted), which comes closer to a needle prick, and finally with a blunt needle (please do not pierce the skin). I use a knitting needle for this purpose. Discuss the procedure with your client beforehand to avoid unpleasant surprises for them.

+++ End of Instructions +++

You can overcome the fear of needles today and let it go ... ... This is easiest when you gradually approach the idea and feeling of an injection while remaining calm ... ... In trance, this is possible ... ... Step by step, it is possible ... ... You already know how it works, but now it is time to experience it ... ... Now, it is really time to stay calm with injections ... ... Your body simply relearns ... ... Your whole body is now learning for you how to stay calm with injections ... ... to experience injections as a normal feeling

… … in calmness … … free from fear and in calmness … … free from fear and in calmness … …

+++ First Stimulus Presentation (Lightly place a finger on the client's arm) +++

You feel calm and balanced now … … and if you think you should feel even more comfortable or it should be even more convenient, then make yourself as comfortable as possible … … Let your breath flow calmly and evenly, because that way you become calmer inside … … That way, you remain in a beautiful state of calm and relaxation … … It is very easy … … You are calm and relaxed … …

… [Apply the stimulus shortly before saying the word "injection" and then remove it. So, briefly place your finger on the client's arm and remove it when you say the next word.] …

… … You are now relaxed … … You are relaxed when it comes to an injection … … very calm, just like now … … Now, it is even easy to stay calm at the thought of an injection … … very calm … … very good … … Now, it works … … You imagine an injection and remain calm … …

+++ Second Stimulus Presentation (Apply pressure with your finger on the client's arm) +++

Keep breathing calmly and evenly and return completely to calmness … … Relax even deeper and deeper … … very good … … You are and remain relaxed and calm … …

… [Apply the stimulus again shortly before saying the word "injection" and then remove it. Press your finger with a bit of pressure on the client's arm and remove it when you say the next word.] …

… … You are now relaxed … … You are relaxed when it comes to an injection … … very calm, just like now … … Now, it is even easy to stay calm at the thought of an injection … … very calm … … very good … … Now, it works … … You imagine an injection and remain calm … …

+++ Third Stimulus Presentation (Place a pen with the tip retracted on the client's arm) +++

Keep breathing calmly and evenly and return completely to calmness … … Relax even deeper and deeper … … very good … … You are and remain relaxed and calm … …

... [Apply the stimulus again shortly before saying the word "injection" and then remove it. Press the pen briefly on the client's arm and remove it when you say the next word.] ...

... ... You are now relaxed ... ... You are relaxed when it comes to an injection ... ... very calm, just like now ... ... Now, it is even easy to stay calm at the thought of an injection ... ... very calm ... ... very good ... ... Now, it works ... ... You imagine an injection and remain calm ... ...

+++ Fourth Stimulus Presentation (Apply pressure with a knitting needle on the client's arm) +++

Keep breathing calmly and evenly and return completely to calmness ... ... Relax even deeper and deeper ... ... very good ... ... You are and remain relaxed and calm ... ...

... [Apply the stimulus again shortly before saying the word "injection" and then remove it. Briefly press with a blunt needle that does not penetrate the skin (e.g., a knitting needle) on the client's arm and remove it when you say the next word.] ...

... ... You are now relaxed ... ... You are relaxed when it comes to an injection ... ... very calm, just like now ... ...

Now, it is even easy to stay calm at the thought of an injection ... ... very calm ... ... very good ... ... Now, it works ... ... You imagine an injection and remain calm ... ...

Now, there is calmness in you again ... ... Calmness that has connected with the feeling of the injection ... ... Today, you have experienced that the feeling of the needle on your skin can no longer unsettle you ... ... With the feeling of the needle touching and piercing your skin, you remain calm ... ... You have just experienced that the needle touching your skin keeps you calm, because you have remained calm ... ... completely calm ... ... From now on, contact with needles will always bring you into this calm state because your body remembers the next time you get an injection, the calmness you felt today ... ... Injections remind your body of the calmness you feel now ... ...

Hypnosis 8

Instructions for Execution

A self-hypnosis trigger is a signal that initiates the state of trance. With its help, even an inexperienced client can continue to work with self-hypnosis at home. Of course, they can "only" work with simple suggestions that they can easily remember and that we should prepare, or also with simple visualizations. Triggered self-hypnosis is a very good tool to give the client a task and to promote therapy. This way, the time between the appointments in the practice is not without therapy but is continued at home. A completely self-directed self-hypnosis, without a trigger, is also easily learnable, but it requires a lot of time and practice.

Setting up the trigger is quite a simple task and naturally relieves the client, who I do not want to burden with practicing a self-directed self-hypnosis. Despite all the naysayers, I also claim here that it is really no problem to teach a client simple triggered self-hypnosis. It is no more dangerous than meditation, autogenic training, or yoga. You also survive them unharmed at home. I have experienced numerous patients in my practice who not only handled self-hypnosis well but enjoyed it. And if a patient enjoys doing self-hypnosis, no matter how simple the suggestion may seem, then it is a very good support for compliance. Discuss the process once before hypnosis and give the client a short, keyword list of the steps of self-hypnosis so that they have a little guide.

+++ End of Instructions +++

Today, I will show you and practice with you how to do self-hypnosis ... ... With self-hypnosis, you can easily work every day to become more and more relaxed ... ... You can actively work on further letting go of your fear of injections until the next session ... ... The good thing is that in a few moments, through the suggestions you hear, you will already let go of a large part of the fear ... ... and feel relaxation and confidence again ... ... Relaxation and confidence in contact with injections ... ... And at the same time, you learn how to do hypnosis with yourself ... ... It is easier than you think ... ...

For this, it is now important that you concentrate on the trance you are in right now ... ... Consciously feel the deep relaxation within you ... ... Now ... ... Consciously feel the calmness within you ... ... Now ... ...

Self-hypnosis is easy if you prepare for it here and now ... ... You need a simple trigger ... ... This is a special word that leads you into trance ... ... It is really simple ... ... The word is ... ... Ridola ... [Emphasize the made-up word by stressing the "Ri" ... Ri-dola.] ... ...

In self-hypnosis, you enter a beautiful trance, just like here ... ... and you are in absolute safety while doing so ... ... Simply make yourself comfortable at home and whisper your self-hypnosis word over and over again until you become tired ... ...

So, whisper ... ... Ridola – Ridola – Ridola – Ridola – Ridola ... ... and in doing so, you automatically enter a beautiful trance ... ... perhaps just as deep as here ... ... But it is enough to enter a very light trance ... ... Your subconscious now deeply imprints the self-hypnosis word Ridola ... ... From now on, you can use this word to enter trance ... ... As soon as you whisper it with closed eyes, you go into trance ... ...

Then you deepen your trance a bit by whispering ten times ... ... I sink deeper and deeper into trance ... ... You simply whisper ... ... I sink once deeper and deeper into trance ... ... I sink twice deeper and deeper into trance ... ... I sink three times deeper and deeper into trance ... ... and so on ... ... until you soon reach ten and whisper ... ... I sink ten times deeper and deeper into trance ... ... With these words that you whisper yourself, you really go into trance ... ... A part of you sinks deep into relaxation while another part stays awake enough to continue guiding your self-hypnosis ... ... You are in complete safety while doing so ... ...

Then comes the main part, the most important part of your self-hypnosis ... ... Now, it is about letting go of fear and building a good feeling with injections ... ... You whisper a suggestion ten times ... ... Ten times you whisper ... ... I feel absolutely comfortable with injections ... ... Again, you count as you do this ... ... Whisper ... ... I feel absolutely comfortable with injections once ... ... I feel absolutely comfortable with injections twice ... ... I feel absolutely comfortable with injections three times ... ... and finally ... ... I feel absolutely comfortable with injections ten times ... ... That is enough then

… … Perhaps you have noticed that these suggestions are already helping you now … … Already now, your fear is dissolving, and you feel comfortable … … and with each repetition in self-hypnosis, you feel more comfortable … …

Waking up after self-hypnosis is easy because you are already awake in hypnosis … … You only need to redirect your attention outward again … … That is how it is here too … … Imagine waking up by opening a window, it becomes cold in the room, and you look outside … … And then you say … … I want to go outside again … … and then you quickly count to three and open your eyes … … So, once again … … To wake up, imagine an open window and let it get cold, then say clearly and loudly … … I want to go outside again – One – Two – Three … … and then open your eyes … …

Your subconscious has learned for you to quickly enter the state of trance with your self-hypnosis word … … It is completely safe and easy … … You can try it yourself right away … … You know how it works … … Your self-hypnosis word Ridola puts you into trance … …

You then deepen it with the words I sink deeper and deeper into trance ... ... Then comes your suggestion ... I feel absolutely comfortable with injections ...

... ... And then you imagine an open window and the cold and say ... I want to go outside again – One – Two – Three ... ... Then you are awake and open your eyes ... ...

Hypnosis 9

You are ready to let go of your fear once and for all today ... ... You have decided ... ... You are ready to take this step ... ... You know that the fear of needles and injections no longer serves any purpose ... ... It is no longer part of your life ... ... You have decided to leave it behind ... ... Because it no longer has any significance ... ... You know this fear well ... ... But now it is in the past ... ... It is over ... ... truly over ... ... You are making a shift ... ... You are shifting your thoughts ... ... to relaxation ... ... Relaxation with needles and injections ... ... You are shifting your feelings ... ... to relaxation ... ... Relaxation with needles and injections ... ... You have already made the shift ... ... You have already taken this step of change internally ... ... Today, you take it for your waking life ... ... From today on, you can also handle needles and injections with ease while awake ... ... As soon as you are fully awake again ... ... you will be free ... ...

When your mind thinks about the fear of injections ... ... then you quickly realize ... ... that it is unfounded ... ... It was an exaggerated fear ... ... that you can now influence with your thoughts … … You can change it … … Because thoughts can amplify fears … … or let them go … … because at some point, you judged a concern or uncertainty too harshly … … But today, you are changing your thinking … … Today, you are making it clear to yourself … … that a small needle cannot harm you at all … … that a small needle does not even hurt … … It just gives you a small pinch … … So, you simply think … … Needles do not matter to me at all … … You might still doubt this … … but in a few moments it will be so … … Perhaps it is already the case … … because in this deep relaxation, needles really do not matter to you at all … …

You feel the calmness of your body … … because you are now in this beautiful state of deep calm … … truly deep calm … … Now, it is also easy to recognize … … that your body is in complete safety … … You are completely safe here … … Nothing can happen to you or your body now … … and now you can also imagine … … that a small prick is no problem at all for your body … … A small sting is just as insignificant … … Surely, you have been bitten by a mosquito before … … and felt a little prick … … no big deal … … actually not a problem at all … … Your body easily handles it … … Your body can now adjust even more … … to experiencing a small prick as insignificant … … to considering the prick of a small needle as insignificant … … insignificant needles … … insignificant pricks … … insignificant little sting … …

Body and feelings are closely connected … … A calm and relaxed body helps you … … to be calm internally as well … … It even makes you automatically calm inside … … You are experiencing that right now … … Because your body is relaxed … … relaxed in deep trance … … you are also relaxed inside … … relaxed in your feelings … … You feel calmness and serenity within you … … you can now even think calmly about injections … … and still remain calm and serene … … because your body is helping you … … because your body is helping you now and will help you in your waking state as well … … And now it is completely clear to you … … that your body hardly registers a small needle prick … … Your body smiles at a small needle prick … … And when you get an injection … … it is again the case … … that your body can laugh about it … … It hardly feels it … … and it does not care … … and this feeling is now clearly passed on to your thoughts by your body … … Then it also does not matter to you in your thoughts … … to see a needle … …

There are even more connections between body and feelings ... ... There is the special connection between action, body, and feelings ... ... Just as your body sensations influence your emotions, so your actions influence your body ... ... and therefore your feelings as well ... ... It is very simple ... ... At the beginning of the trance, you experienced ... ... that you calmed down through actions ... ... You made yourself comfortable ... ... You closed your eyes ... ... and you breathed slowly and evenly ... ... You are still doing that ... ... and exactly that helped your body ... ... to enter this beautiful state of deep relaxation ... ... and to stay there ... ... This also works in your everyday life ... ... Conscious calm breathing calms your body ... ... keeps your heartbeat calm ... ... and as a result, you feel emotionally relaxed ... ... free from any fear ... ... and full of peace ... ... free from fear and full of peace ... ... peace that makes you serene ... ... and needles do not matter to you ... ... Needles are completely indifferent to you ... ... Needles are truly indifferent to you ... ...

You have come much closer to your goal today ... ... because you have already changed your basic attitude towards needles and injections ... ... You have changed more than you might think ... ... You have realized that it was a completely exaggerated fear ... ... that had taken hold of you ... ... You have adjusted your thoughts ... ... have taken to heart the thought ... ... that tells you ... ... Needles do not matter to me at all ... ... first as an idea ... ... as a wish ... ... But today, in trance ... ... this wish has sunk deeper ... ... and become a truth ... ... Your body has remained calm ... ... You have remained calm inside ... ... calm in the thought of needles and injections ... ... and this calmness remains ... ... because you will always be able to stay calm ... ... and remain calm with injections ... ... Needles do not matter to you at all ... ... You just keep breathing naturally ... ... calmly breathing in and out ... ... free from fear and full of peace ... ... truly free from fear and full of peace ... ...

Hypnosis 10

Deep in trance, you can imagine more than in the waking state ... ... Now, you can imagine more than in the waking state, because in this beautiful calmness, your imagination can move much more freely and openly ... ... Imagination is something that lies within all of us ... ... and imagination is also what you can use today to free yourself from fear ... ... The world of imagination has a name ... ... It is like an inexhaustible reservoir of ideas and thoughts ... ... Imagination is like a land you can travel to ... ... The land of dreams ... ... Dream and reality ... ... Often, we think they are two different worlds, but both are real, and both are equally important ... ... and both are always there ... ... Your attention decides where you are ... ... and now you direct your attention inward ... ... and you go into the land of dreams ... ...

You are standing in a large meadow and looking out over the land ... ... As far as your eye can see, you can see blooming nature ... ... Everything here appears in harmony ... ... You see vast fields and meadows ... ... Forests with mighty, ancient trees … … and huge mountains in the background that rise from the beautiful land and reach up to the sky … … Rivers flow through the land, and on the water of the rivers, the sunlight sparkles and breaks … … You look up … … The sky is bright and clear … … and cloudless … … It is a beautiful summer day … … A warm wind blows over the land of dreams and invites you to let go of your thoughts … … It is as if the wind is carrying your thoughts away … … You start walking, strolling leisurely through the meadow, and enjoying the calmness in the land of dreams … … Your thoughts become free and light, for the warm wind is indeed carrying them away … … In the land of dreams, you never have to think … … Everything that wants to be seen shows itself on its own in images and feelings … … It is enough to let all the images and feelings be … … That is enough … …

… … Then suddenly, it is as if you have walked very far, even though you are strolling so calmly and have walked step by step without a goal … … But in the land of dreams, you do not need a goal, for you always find the same thing … … Here, you always find yourself … … whatever you are looking for … … You find yourself … … Then you see a huge field, made up entirely of red roses … … a rose field with roses without thorns … … In the land of dreams, roses never have thorns … … You come to the field and just keep walking … … You walk through the field, and with your fingertips, you touch the petals of the roses … … They feel so delicate and fine … … The roses are very delicate … … like silk … … You remember that red roses are the flowers of love … … People in love give each other red roses … … But in the land of dreams, love primarily means self-love … … because everything here is always a part of you … … So, the rose field is also a part of you … … the part that can love yourself … … the part of you that can love yourself even when you are afraid … … even when you are afraid of needles or afraid of injections … … Maybe you think you could not love yourself for that because in your mind and thoughts, you have judged yourself or thought it was abnormal to have such a fear … … But the land of dreams tells you that fear is a normal reaction … .. .a reaction that is like an overload … … Too often in your life, you have cared more about others than about yourself … … often, you simply had too little time for yourself … … That is how it happened that many feelings have remained within you … … and over time, these feelings sought a way to be seen after all ... ... They broke out as fear ... ... Originally, it might not have even been fear ... ... There were many feelings that you could not see ... ... It was not your fault, you often simply did not have the time or opportunity to deal with them ... ... You would have needed someone to help you, just as you have often helped others ... ...

... ... You keep walking through the field and think about how the thorns of life have often pricked or stabbed you ... ... Many times, you have taken the stabs, perhaps you could not defend yourself ... ... because you might have been too young ... ... or because no one helped you ... ... Your memory returns ... ... Perhaps there were some big and deep stabs you experienced ... ... Disappointments ... ... maybe betrayal ... ... And then there were certainly many small stabs ... ... Individually and by themselves, you could endure them ... ... You kept going, even when it hurt ... ... Eventually, the pain lessened, and you might have thought then that you had overcome or processed the stabs ... ... But in reality, you had only gotten used to the pain ... ... You remember ... ... there were these stabs ... ... big and small ... ... the stabs of life ... ... thorns and needles of life ... ... and over time, it became too much ... ... so much that your entire inner self rebels against further stabs ... ... against pricks ... ... against deep stabs ... ... Your body shows it to you ... ... It has reacted to stabs, to needles and injections, with fear ... ... But it actually shows you that deep inside, you are no longer willing to take the stabs of life ... ... because they are not fate ... ... Stabs were inflicted on you ... ... The land of dreams tells you on your way through the rose field without thorns that deep inside, you thought it had to be that way ... ... Maybe you also thought it was right that you were being punished ... ... because you had heard something similar from other people ... ... You pick a few roses and take them with you on your way to your waking everyday life ... ... You give yourself the flowers of love ... ... Love from you to you ... ... Love from you to you ... ...

You reach the edge of the field ... ... You continue walking across a meadow and find a beautiful spot where you can rest ... ... in the middle of the sun or in the shade of a tree, just as you like ... ... You rest ... ... no more thorns ... ... no more stabs ... ... You are allowed to defend yourself against stabs and pricks ... ... The land of dreams gives you love ... ... with your self-love, which frees you from every fear in your waking everyday life ... ... Why does this happen? ... ...

Because the land of dreams is not a fairy tale ... ... it is truth ... ... the truth of your feelings ... ... You think about the fact that the land of dreams lies deep within you ... ... It has always been there ... ... I am just telling you about it ... ...

Distribution, publication, and copying in any form are prohibited and subject to damages.

All Titles in the Series

Volume 1: Smoking Cessation
Volume 2: Anxiety and Restlessness
Volume 3: Burnout
Volume 4: Reducing Overweight
Volume 5: Coping with the Past
Volume 6: Suicidal Thoughts and Attempts
Volume 7: Psycho-Oncology
Volume 8: Obsessions and Tics
Volume 9: Self-Confidence and Decision-Making
Volume 10: Grief Work
Volume 11: Psychosomatics
Volume 12: Chronic Pain
Volume 13: Depressive Thoughts
Volume 14: Panic Attacks
Volume 15: Domestic Violence, Victim Support
Volume 16: Post-Traumatic Stress
Volume 17: Exam Anxiety and Stage Fright
Volume 18: Anti-Violence Training, Offender Support
Volume 19: Addiction Tendencies
Volume 20: Social Phobia and Fear of Contact
Volume 21: Nail Biting
Volume 22: Self-Awareness and Self-Love
Volume 23: Teeth Grinding and Night Clenching
Volume 24: Feelings of Guilt
Volume 25: Fear in Crowds
Volume 26: Fear of Flying, Aviophobia
Volume 27: Fear in Enclosed Spaces, Claustrophobia
Volume 28: Tinnitus, Ear Noises
Volume 29: Fear of Heights
Volume 30: Neurodermatitis

Copying, publishing, and sharing with third parties are only permitted with the written consent of the author. Please observe the notes on copyright and usage.

Volume 31: Finding Inner Balance
Volume 32: Overcoming Loneliness
Volume 33: Fear of Illness, Hypochondria
Volume 34: Anticipatory Anxiety, Fear of Fear
Volume 35: Jealousy in Relationships
Volume 36: Driving Anxiety
Volume 37: New Start after Separation
Volume 38: Fear of Injections
Volume 39: Heart Anxiety Neurosis
Volume 40: Overcoming Resentment and Anger
Volume 41: Resolving Blockages and Positive Thinking
Volume 42: Stress Reduction, Stress Management
Volume 43: Body Relaxation
Volume 44: Deep Relaxation
Volume 45: Fear of the Dark
Volume 46: Falling Asleep and Staying Asleep
Volume 47: Compulsive Buying
Volume 48: Restless Legs Syndrome
Volume 49: Bulimia
Volume 50: Anorexia
Volume 51: Overcoming Nightmares
Volume 52: Imagined Deformity
Volume 53: Overcoming Distrust, Finding Trust
Volume 54: Processing Failures
Volume 55: Humiliation, Emotional Hurt
Volume 56: Distressing Compassion, Vicarious Suffering
Volume 57: Self-Forgiveness
Volume 58: Self-Awareness, Self-Confidence
Volume 59: Saying No
Volume 60: Assertiveness
Volume 61: Setting Boundaries and Self-Assertion
Volume 62: Decision-Making Ability

Volume 63: Success Orientation
Volume 64: Ruminating, Circular Thinking
Volume 65: Accepting Pregnancy
Volume 66: Birth Preparation
Volume 67: Spiritual Opening
Volume 68: Joy of Life and Inner Lightness
Volume 69: Patience and Inner Peace
Volume 70: Fibromyalgia and Rheumatism
Volume 71: Irritable Bowel Syndrome, Crohn's Disease
Volume 72: Fear of Nausea, Emetophobia
Volume 73: Stuttering and Cluttering, Speech Flow Disorders
Volume 74: Concentration and Knowledge Anchoring
Volume 75: Vitality and Spontaneity
Volume 76: Searching for Meaning and Finding Goals
Volume 77: Life Crises, Life Events
Volume 78: Workaholism, Goal Obsession
Volume 79: Helper Syndrome, Helpless Helpers
Volume 80: Medication Abuse
Volume 81: Gambling Addiction
Volume 82: Internet Addiction, Smartphone Addiction
Volume 83: Hoarding Disorder, Compulsive Collecting
Volume 84: Conspiracy Thoughts, Overvalued Ideas
Volume 85: Fear of Operations and Treatments
Volume 86: Fear of Aging
Volume 87: Travel Anxiety
Volume 88: Anxiety When Urinating, Paruresis
Volume 89: Fear of Intimacy and Togetherness
Volume 90: Fear of Blushing
Volume 91: Coming Out in Homosexuality
Volume 92: Charisma Training
Volume 93: Migraines and Chronic Headaches
Volume 94: Overcoming Allergies, Bronchial Asthma

Volume 95: Normalizing Blood Pressure
Volume 96: Compulsive Perfectionism
Volume 97: Sports Hypnosis, Motivation
Volume 98: Sports Hypnosis, Performance Enhancement
Volume 99: Determination and Focus
Volume 100: Encountering the Inner Child
Volume 101: Cravings, Binge Eating
Volume 102: Stimulating Metabolism
Volume 103: Bipolar Mood Swings
Volume 104: Borderline, Identity Crises
Volume 105: Hypomania, Euphoria, Mania
Volume 106: Restlessness, Agitation
Volume 107: Nervous Breakdown
Volume 108: Adjustment Disorders
Volume 109: Self-Alienation, Depersonalization
Volume 110: Ending Self-Pity
Volume 111: Primary Gain of Illness
Volume 112: Secondary Gain of Illness
Volume 113: Bullying, Victim Support
Volume 114: Letting Go of Envy and Jealousy
Volume 115: Fear of Spiders, Arachnophobia
Volume 116: Fear of Dogs or Cats
Volume 117: Fear of Strangers, Xenophobia
Volume 118: Excessive Worries, Generalized Anxiety
Volume 119: Strengthening Sense of Responsibility
Volume 120: Unrequited Love, Heartache
Volume 121: Work-Life Balance
Volume 122: Letting Go of Unattainable Goals
Volume 123: Allowing and Accepting Help
Volume 124: Letting Go of Adult Children
Volume 125: Tourette Syndrome
Volume 126: Life Changes and New Starts

Volume 127: Accepting Life in a Wheelchair
Volume 128: Understanding and Overcoming Homesickness
Volume 129: Understanding and Overcoming Wanderlust
Volume 130: Dizziness, Meniere's Disease
Volume 131: Overcoming Aggression
Volume 132: Cutting and Self-Harm
Volume 133: Hair Pulling, Trichotillomania
Volume 134: Postpartum Depression
Volume 135: For Relatives of Dementia Patients
Volume 136: Self-Harm, Artificial Disorders
Volume 137: Activating Self-Healing Powers
Volume 138: Preventing Depression Relapse
Volume 139: Reactive Psychoses, Follow-Up
Volume 140: Obsessive Thoughts and Impulses
Volume 141: Compulsive Checking
Volume 142: Compulsive Counting, Symmetry Obsession
Volume 143: Compulsive Washing, Cleanliness Obsession
Volume 144: Compulsive Questioning
Volume 145: Dissociative Paralysis
Volume 146: Phantom Pain
Volume 147: Overcoming Complaining
Volume 148: Hay Fever, Pollen Allergy
Volume 149: Sexual Abuse, Victim Support
Volume 150: Standing Strong Against Sexism, #metoo
Volume 151: Binge Eating
Volume 152: Overcoming Thoughts of Revenge
Volume 153: Detachment from the Aggressor, Stockholm Syndrome
Volume 154: Courage to Separate
Volume 155: Chronic Fatigue, Exhaustion
Volume 156: Fear of the Future, Existential Anxiety
Volume 157: Excessive Worry About Children
Volume 158: Fear of Failure

Volume 159: Ending Distrust and Control
Volume 160: Dejection, Dysphoria
Volume 161: Boreout, Chronic Boredom
Volume 162: Bipolar Disorders, Relapse Prevention
Volume 163: Mania, Relapse Prevention
Volume 164: Nihilism, Feelings of Worthlessness
Volume 165: Thumb Sucking
Volume 166: Being Brave
Volume 167: Being Proud
Volume 168: Overcoming Shyness
Volume 169: Being Able to Delegate Responsibility
Volume 170: Being Able to Show Emotions
Volume 171: Letting Go of Guilt, Victim Support
Volume 172: Processing Guilt, Offender Support
Volume 173: Mood Swings, Cyclothymia
Volume 174: Lack of Drive, Vital Sadness
Volume 175: Hearing Voices with Reality Reference
Volume 176: Confident Communication
Volume 177: Standing Up for Oneself
Volume 178: Taking New Paths
Volume 179: Confident Job Application
Volume 180: No Longer Being Taken Advantage Of
Volume 181: End of Submissiveness
Volume 182: Depressive Numbness
Volume 183: Mood Drops, Affective Incontinence
Volume 184: Mood Instability
Volume 185: Somatoform Disorders
Volume 186: Stomach Ulcer, Psychosomatic
Volume 187: Accepting Amputation
Volume 188: Overcoming and Letting Go of Hatred
Volume 189: Ending Accusations
Volume 190: Allowing Tears, Being Able to Cry

Volume 191: Finding and Sorting Repressed Feelings
Volume 192: Somatoform Pain
Volume 193: Living Autonomously
Volume 194: Anhedonia, Joylessness
Volume 195: Persistent Sadness
Volume 196: Obesity, Food Addiction
Volume 197: Parents of Abused Children
Volume 198: Letting Go and Letting Be
Volume 199: Childhood Sexual Abuse
Volume 200: Fear of Loss

www.ingramcontent.com/pod-product-compliance
Lightning Source LLC
Chambersburg PA
CBHW030501220526
45464CB00006B/2605